Legal notice

Pictures & illustrations:

Most of the pictures and illustrations published have been designed from Canva

Book cover designed by Francoise Foulet

This page intentionally left blank

Are we ready to manage our health in the metaverse?

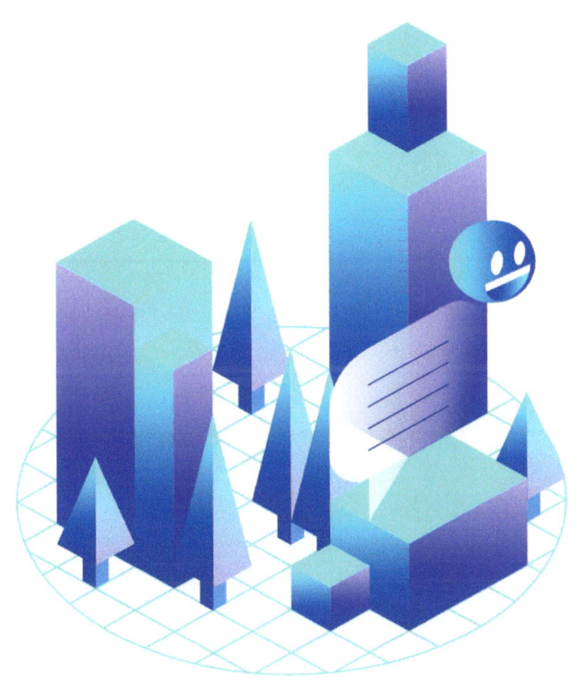

Quotes from top talents in AI, Metaverse and Blockchain

Part 1

Dr Luc Julia, Innovator & Siri's co-founder (*Apple*)

"Metaverse helps us to simulate the real into the virtual world"

Part 2

Michael Kaldasch, CEO of *Aimedis*

"There is no definition of virtual or meta-hospital!"

Dr Alain Perez, Hospital surgeon & Author

"We have to demystify the hospital by using the virtual world to prepare the patient before to be treated in the real life"

Part 3

Oleg Fomenko, Co-founder of *Sweatcoin*

"The biggest challenge that I see is to create a working economy with changing inputs to achieve an optimal balance between users motivation to move and growth"

Part 4

Philippe Gerwill, Advisory board member at *DeHealth*

"Metaverse needs much more education. It's not just gaming. We need new blood, to bring this thing to pharma"

Part 5

Weronika Marciniak, Metaverse Architect at *Future is Meta*

"For the daylife. I think metaverse is the future of internet. There is no reason to believe that metaverse isn't accessible for fragile people"

Dr Luc Julia, Innovator & Siri's co-founder (*Apple*)

"Metaverse dedicated to Alzheimer would be interesting!"

INTRODUCTION

This short essay is a reflection, and immersion, into the virtual world known as the metaverse. To keep from boring you, the 5 stories presented here will be a mix of reality and fiction. We will see that the metaverse could change a lot of things in healthcare such as, the way we are treated, the way we live our patient or doctor experience and the entire lucrative market behind healthcare.

Before starting, it is necessary to give a little definition of what the metaverse is. The metaverse is a virtual world that is a continuation of the real world. In the virtual world that everybody calls the metaverse, everyone is able to work, make friends, buy land on *Decentraland* or also see a doctor in a 3D hospital. The number of users is unlimited and they may be in the form of a robot, animal or simply in their purest appearance. The metaverse is a digital environment, which implements virtual (VR) and augmented-reality (AR) where users can interact with one another in real time.

According to its Greek etymology *meta* means "after something" or "beyond something". As for *verse*, this is simply a contraction of universe. Therefore, the metaverse is this new form of world that comes after the current one.

In 2022, the neologism metaverse is becoming a buzzword. I've participated in a lot of events, workshops and discussions where companies, but also the "man on the street" have used this term. Everyone has their own representation when it comes to the metaverse and, in my opinion, such flagship projects in blockchain and crypto like *Meta* (*Facebook*), *The Sandbox* or *Decentraland* have played an important role in shaping these representations. The current metaverse is based on blockchain which is a technology that is able to store and manage information without a middleman or one central authority. This is the famous case of bitcoin.

In the meanwhile, we are gradually moving from a 2D internet (mail, website, chat, image…) to a 3D internet which is embodied by the metaverse. In other words, the metaverse is the 3D elevation of the current internet. It covers unprecedented virtual simulations in the world around us (augmented reality) and may become a large part of the leisure and consumer socialization.

But as we are going to see, the metaverse is a very promising technology for the future of healthcare. This technology will change the way we experience health and well-being; whether we are a patient, consumer, sportman, doctor, student or nurse.

Medical training is gradually being integrated into the metaverse. Our genetic information will probably be transformed into what we call a Non-Fongible Token (NFT) that could then be sold or used as a proof of identity in the metaverse. Soon, in the metaverse, charity organizations could also receive donations.

According to the consulting firm InsightAce Analytic, the metaverse in the healthcare market may reach USD 71.97 billion by 2030. It is 14 times more than its current market size which was estimated to be USD 5.06 billion in 2021!

The present book is not addressed to a well-defined group of readers. "Real Health, Virtual World" is for everyone and I hope it will inspire entrepreneurs, decision makers and any type of curious person. The book will be split into chapters with two subsections. The first subsection will share a fictional tale about the metaverse, digital assets, decentralized solutions and of course healthcare. Following on a second subsection will focus on strategy and prospective for companies and people willing to conduct research and make business.

Let's explore this virtual healthcare world!

1 – Is immortality possible in the metaverse?

When we talk about the metaverse we will inevitably have to consider it with a touch of fantasy! From time immemorial humans have feared and reckoned with death. That's why, we think or believe that death is an illusion or an issue which we can solve. The field of immortality, for now, also contains an element of fantasy, despite the fact some researchers work on the biology of ageing. These researchers study human and animal cells and their processes of senescence to better understand the biological clock in order to act directly on it.

1.1 – The story of Melinda

The first story I would like to tell you is maybe the most fantastic one. This is the story of a young woman called Melinda who was very concerned about her age. Obviously, we need not disclose Melinda's age as one should never share a women's age! However, Melinda wasn't on the same page. She did not want to get old.

One day when she was checking her phone a notification captured her attention. It was an advert that offered her a chance to create her own avatar for free on *Meta Long life*. At last, she would join the virtual world.

The concept seemed interesting and Melinda was very enthusiastic about the idea of being the same person in reality but also the virtual world. Nevertheless a lot of questions came to mind. How exactly would it work? Would it really be free? What would be the purpose of having a version of oneself in the metaverse?

On *Meta Long Life* accessing the basic virtual world was simple. You just had to create a realistic avatar by scanning your face with your smartphone or laptop cam. A high-resolution camera would be the best to perfectly design ones' skin tone and texture. From there, you would then have the possibility to accept your virtual version, or not.

Meta Long Life was a freemium model, which meant that basic access was free for a limited time period. Melinda would only be able to navigate this virtual world of meeting other people, and accessing different marketplaces (art, apartment, luxurious penthouse…) with little room for development and upgrade. But it didn't matter because this first immersion was very engaging for Melinda and she planning to take further advantage of additional services more focused on health and wellness.

As for a paid version, there were many wonderful opportunities. First of all, for a monthly subscription fee of $50 each newcomer received either a headset, or connected glasses, or lenses equipped with VR or AR technology. After choosing her elegant and comfortable connected glasses she was poised to start a better immersive experience through her avatar. Through the paid version the avatar would automatically convert into an NFT, a unique title of property in this virtual world. Two choices were available either you could sell a piece of yourself on an NFT art platform to directly make money, or you could sell it at a later date hoping that your avatar would be worth more. Once the avatar was matched with a potential buyer Melinda could sell a part of her digital twin and get a token that could be converted into dollars. Besides, the paid version offered features that were very beneficial, especially in terms of health, wellness and cosmetics. For instance, Melinda had an average discount of 10% towards a partner insurer or 50% off if she went with *Meta Long Life insurance*. The reason why she had such a significant reduction was due to the fact that her avatar was collecting personal data in real time. This personal data included: the number of steps she took per day, her frequency of doctor visits, what she had eaten in reality and what she had eaten in the virtual world. Alongside this affordable insurance Melinda had to wear her glasses a minimum of 5 hours a day. She understood that these data points were collected and processed in real time but saw no reason why she shouldn't share them.

Melinda knew that becoming immortal or at least looking younger also involved cosmetics. That's why, she was very excited when she discovered the new partnership between *Meta Long Life* and a famous French cosmetics brand that she loved. Again and again she was getting discounts to buy real and virtual products from this brand. But one day she was intrigued by an announcement that showcased a program called *"Kill the Death"*.

"Kill the Death" was an anti-ageing program scheduled to start in 2 months. At first, selected participants would have the chance to check their real biological age into the metaverse through a virtual DNA moving in 3D. This biological age would show our real body age, or the metabolic age which would be far more accurate than the number of years since you were born. Imagine yourself watching from your sofa a giant virtual DNA indicating your "real age" second per second. It would certainly be scary at first, but the idea ends up seducing Melinda. The *"Kill the Death"* program would be the first immersive experience offered by *Meta Long Life* that would understand that our biological age is very often lower than our chronological age as a result of our lifestyle and genetics. Smoking, drinking, sugar, lack of physical activity and high levels of stress are crucial factors that reduce a person's lifespan. To predict Melinda's ageing a DNA test which analyzed more than 50 000 biomarkers across a person's genome would be sent to her. After receiving this at-home DNA test kit the 25-year-old woman had to collect a saliva sample with a swab and then she simply had to wait a few seconds. After that, she put the swab into a tiny device, which would upload her genetic data directly in the metaverse. Most surprisingly, her avatar seemed to be a little bit younger than her real age at 22 years old as opposed to 25! Melinda didn't realize yet but her own genes related to skin elasticity and inflammatory response had been analyzed in order to determine a cellular ageing. In addition, she thought it was pretty cool she could virtually watch her own biological clock. In order to motivate people to keep a healthy lifestyle the *"Kill the Death"* program would create personalized nutrition and physical activity plans that would then be shared to participants in the metaverse. As *Meta Long Life* is on blockchain and generates its own token called MLL Token *"Kill the Death"* participants would receive a reward in order to purchase real or virtual sport sessions with a coach. Alongside this, they could also access learning content about regenerative medicine and in a second phase participants would get priority access to participate in a clinical trial for rejuvenation therapy. No information was readily available concerning this VIP Access but there were many possibilities to develop specific drugs for age-related diseases, such as, impacting bones (osteoporosis), muscle issues (sarcopenia), and deteriorating vision (wet AMD)...

 In the world of *Meta Long Life* immortality would be possible in both the virtual world and the real world! From calculation age with DNA to rejuvenation therapy, immortality would no longer be a dream thanks to the powers of blockchain and the metaverse. Our genetic data would be stored on blockchain for eternity and for this reason one part of our identity would always be immortalized. Years after her death, Melinda's personal information would be saved and available, albeit in a virtual reality space. More than a utopia, the survival of Melinda's information on a blockchain-based metaverse could also have an impact on what she bequeaths in her inheritance for instance. After her death, Melinda's avatar could reunite with her family and communicate all the necessary details related to her succession. All the virtual and real properties, lands and artworks would be allocated to the relevant beneficiaries, such as, children and grandchildren. This transfer of property could be automated through a program called "Smart Contract" which would be able to automatically perform contract conditions regarding the will of the deceased, in this case, Melinda. What would be even more amazing is that close relatives and friends would have the possibility to communicate with Melinda's digital twin, her avatar, who would not only act like her, but who would also look like her. An AI-driven 3D avatar that mimicked the character of Melinda could offer support and comfort to those living. Even after Melinda's death, artificial intelligence (AI) would ensure that a continuing avatar could have freewill! Let's consider an avatar's freewill and consciousness. Could an AI exist after a real person's death? This idea is maybe one of the biggest challenges the metaverse and it's digital twins are facing up to now.

1.2 – The future of a Human Digital Twin

Before defining what a human digital twin is, I would like to tell my dear readers that the following part will primarily focus on existing and very concrete use cases regarding scientific evolution and discoveries. The primary purpose is to propose ideas for future technological and business developments.

Definition

Globally a digital twin is a virtual representation of a human object or system that might exist in a metaverse. It can be a replica of an object, such as, sports shoes, however it can also be a replica of a human and all its attributes (organs, bones, muscles, DNA, etc.). Every step, every disease, every eating behavior can be updated in real-time to make the right decision at the right time regarding our mental and physical health. Sensors and other kinds of connected objects can synchronize our physical world to the digital world. Any changes, any movements in the material world can be directly reflected in a digital format through our twin. A digital twin is not just a replica of our face or our body. It could be a replica of our heart, femur, brain, bones, muscle, DNA or our entire cardiovascular system. This avatar can reproduce our outer shape, our face or even just one specific organ as a model which could be updated in real-time due to a mobile app making facial analysis, exams, scans and collecting all sorts of data related to our health and general well-being. A human digital twin would be a key part of customized and personalized medicine, but would not be the only benefit!

Use cases & opportunities

Applicability for medicine

The doctor who will be navigating in a metaverse will have a greater freedom to treat his patient. Before a medical appointment, the doctor would register and access a health metaverse. Just typing the name of his patient or his identification number the "Meta Doctor" would be able to visualize one specific part of his patient. Scrolling, zooming and a lot of haptic and tactile functions would be a new routine for the "Meta Doctor". DNA information, molecular profiling, data imaging and data from a patient record would be checked. Doctors could simulate medical interventions such as surgery directly on certain organs merely by watching. Test scenarios would be possible in order to reduce drastically the risk of medical error. Using these test scenarios the specialist could plan their surgery. After surgery the patient's evolution could easily be continuously monitored in the metaverse. Medicine has the opportunity to be completely changed if, and only if, there is a real uptake in the use and adoption of metaverse from doctors and patients.

Metaverse is a way to simulate risk situation where people could imagine vehicle crash-test or an emergency in a nuclear power plant. It is not better to endanger lives in the metaverse? Personally I am for the simulation of emergencies or virtual battlefield medicine in the metaverse rather than real world. We need to think carefully about the creation of patient digital twin! Thanks to the metaverse, we are now able to represent dangerous situations in the automobile sector and in the energy sector. Will the medical sector be the next?

Applicability for the pharmaceutical industry

The following interest is linked to the previous interest of metaverse for medicine. Simulating virtual drug and therapy tests on virtual patients is relevant for both doctors and the pharmaceutical industry. But now, let's consider the pharmaceutical industry. Indeed, the pharmaceutical industry and its contract research organization (CROs) have a great interest to use a metaverse in order to recruit volunteers willing to participate in a clinical trial. Nowadays, we know that more than 60% of patients would be more willing to participate in a clinical trial if their time and travel time were reduced through the use of remote devices, which would benefit from real-time remote monitoring. So here's the bonus of the metaverse! In exchange for compensation we could imagine the metaverse offering the participant a cool and playful environment to participate in a clinical trial via their digital twin. Even if the participant is at home or outside sensors would collect real-time data which could then be transferred to the scientists leading the trial. This would therefore reduce time costs and would accelerate the development time of a drug. In terms of remuneration the pharmaceutical industry would be able to pay the participants directly in their own cryptocurrency (crypto). Let's say a sort of clinical trial token called *CT token*. Once the participant gets their crypto they will be able to convert it to earn more crypto. Then he could pay for goods and services in the metaverse or convert his cryptocurrency as a revenue stream.

Applicability for sport and fitness

 Big sport & sportswear brands seem very interested in the metaverse, as a means to sell more products like shoes, sports clothes, equipment and even the latest sport fashion. These brands know very well that people always want more personalized features for their avatar. Most of them want the latest real sneakers for their own avatar in the metaverse. Beyond this aspect, a digital twin presents a real opportunity in the field of sports biomechanics, which is the science of physics that improves an athlete's sports performance. Researchers all across the world are working in this field, and they use, for instance, hundreds of thousands of images of athletes in a 3D model to compare and match them with a 2D model[1]. Many scans of athletes and sportsmen could be made and compared to two-dimensional models in order to study body fat, bones and muscles density. The metaverse is the perfect area to host a digital twin for sport performance. Let's imagine a metaverse for athletes, where after scanning their movement in a slow motion mode they get simulations based on real data they have given. This

---

[1]   Marcel Rossi, Andrew Lyttle, Amar El-Sallam, Nat Benjanuvatra, Brian Blanksby, *Body Segment Inertial Parameters of elite swimmers Using DXA and indirect Methods,* 2013

simulation in the metaverse could improve specific skills, such as a tennis serve or foot-eye-coordination in football. The metaverse could be the beginning of an extremely lucrative sports training program, which tech sport start-ups and sports brands could use to coach and monitor their athletes. This science of the movement that could be applied through a VR or AR helmet could be able to prevent injury like common knee injury, which is widespread in the world of runners. By analogy, this tech would be important for people suffering functional disabilities such as dependent seniors with difficulties to walk or disabled people. Wearable AI technology and scanning solutions would be crucial to get a high level of accuracy, therefore improving performance, predicting certain types of injury and helping surgeons make best practice decisions.

Applicability for user authentication

As surprising as it may sound, a digital twin, a digital carbon copy of our body and our genetic information presents could be used to prove whom we are like a sort of ID or passport. Indeed, a DNA-based digital twin could be stored on blockchain and would allow us to access personal accounts such as an administrative file, a patient record or a bank account. But how do we proceed? Part of the answer may lie in biometric sensors analyzing in real time many attributes of our body such as sweat. In my opinion genetic data and many personal information related to lifestyle, medical history, nutrition or weight size are conclusive as a piece of evidence. Nowadays, identity systems in a hospital, telehealth platforms or social media are centralized and this leads to a "balkanization of identities", which is why users often create different identities. This is an effect of data silos that gives less control to the user and more control to the online services. Therefore, decentralized identity has a real added-value for the user because no central institution would, or could, hold control over it. Through an NFT we could bring our own identity pass with us everywhere as a proof of identity based on our health information.

Challenges

Despite the many applications of a digital twin across the metaverse, some challenges persist to this day. The first is the importance of sensitivity, which depends on haptic technology, which constantly trying to improve the sense of touch with great accuracy. Avatar and digital twin are also facing a big challenge concerning emotion. Does an avatar think and feel human emotions? To engage more people in a long-term period, businesses have to keep working on feeling and emotion in the metaverse. There is a real competitive advantage to develop this feature when it comes to "human" digital twin and health services. Data only creates value if your company or public entity is able to collect, process, qualify and deliver it in clear and actionable insights. Digital twins play a major role for companies and public bodies that want to transform their data into a powerful performance lever. Data has to be readable and understandable to any type of user, whether experts or not. That's the magic of digital twins for organization! All risks related to physical and verbal abuse, or virtual addiction, have to be taken into account. Finally, there must be regulation on cyber-violence to ensure the metaverse is safe and to make sure it does not attract miscreants or offenders.

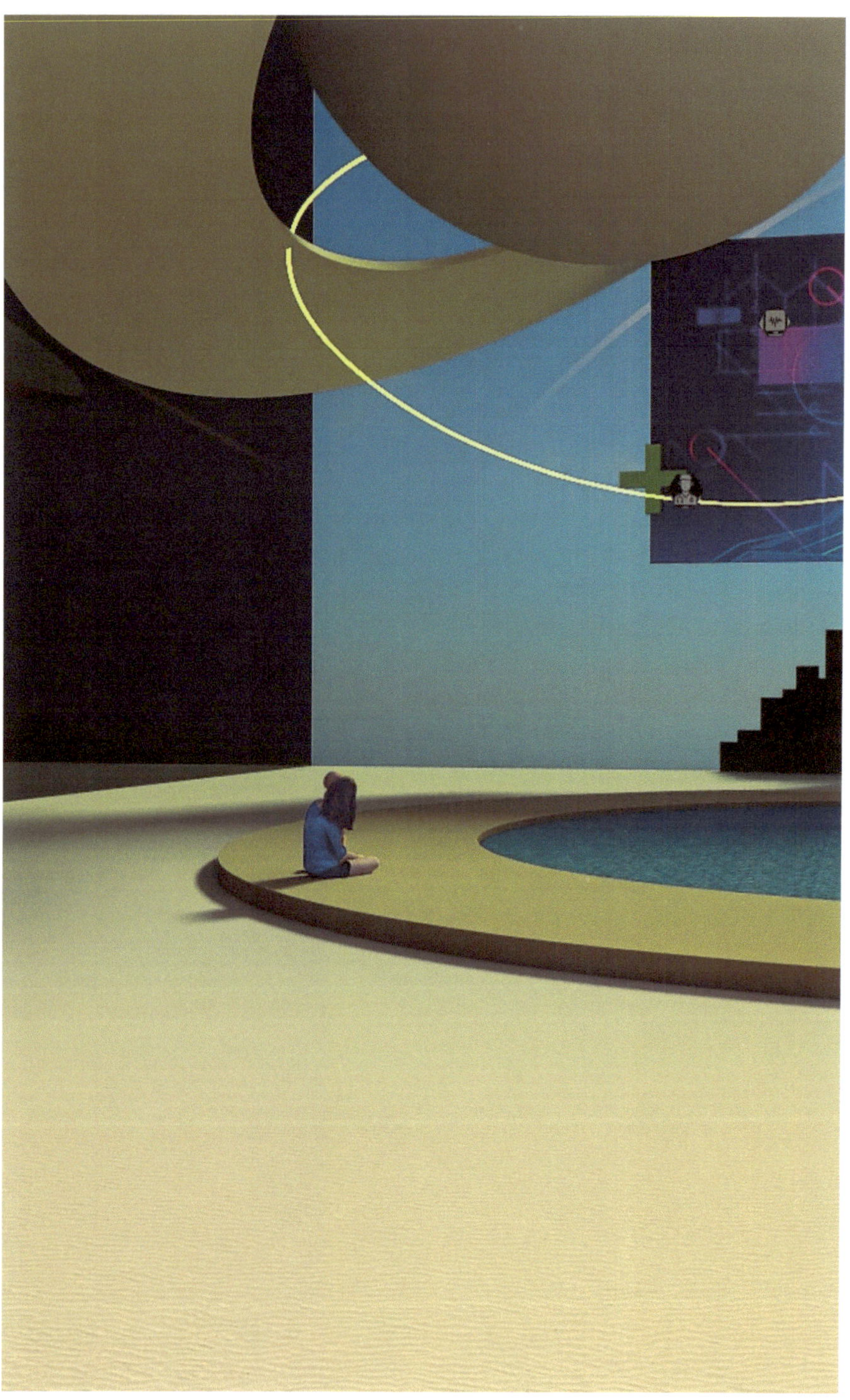

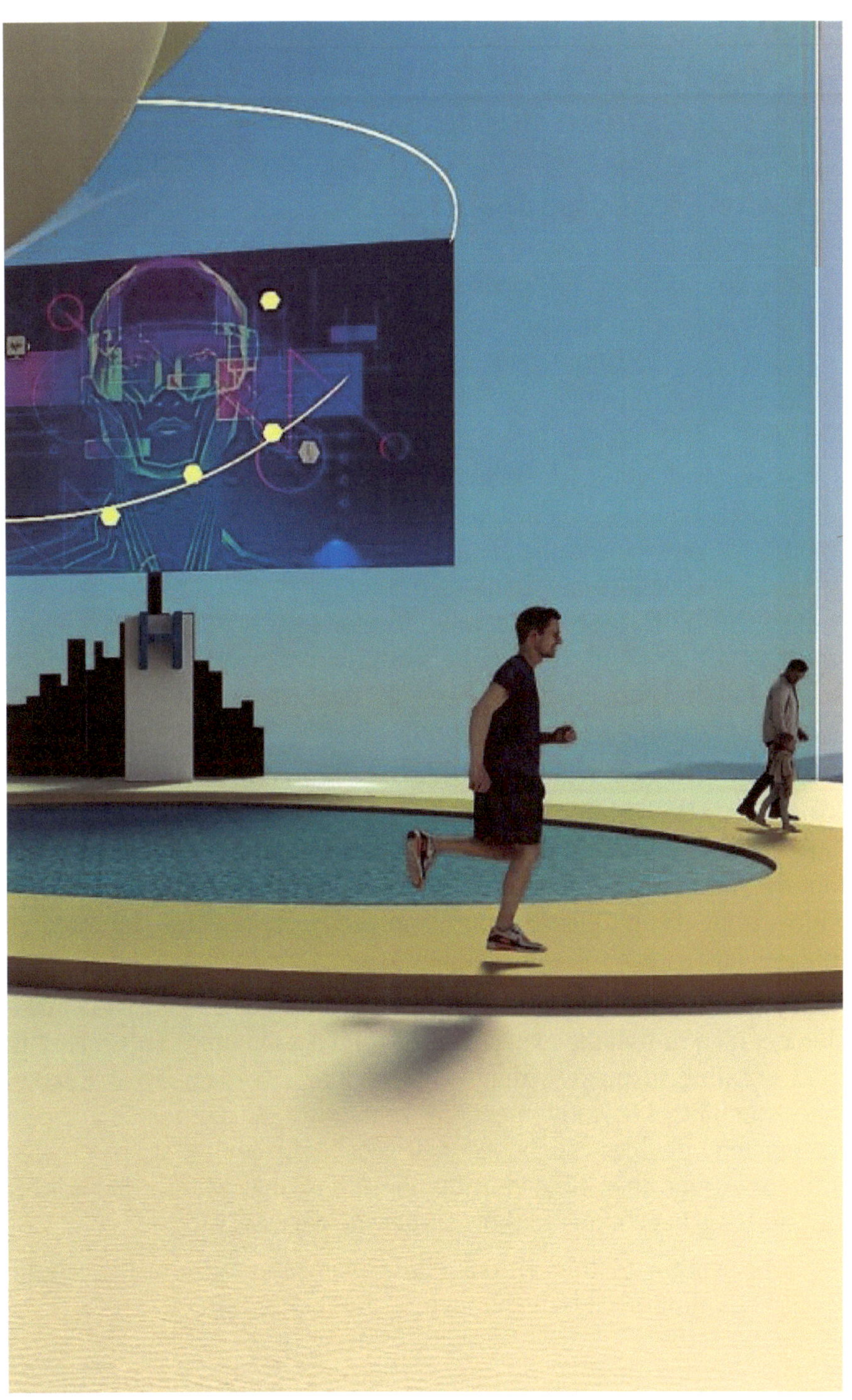

2 – Why do we need hospitals & health services in the virtual world?

2.1 – The story of Joe

Joe was an accomplished sportsman who practiced running, football and tennis several times a week. However for a few months Joe had been feeling a pain when he bent his knees and this had been debilitating, not only for his sport practice, but also for his everyday life.

As a result, it was clear that he needed a medical consultation, in order to find out whether he needed surgery or simply several months of rest. Unfortunately, in the last five years waiting times in general & specialty medicine have increased. Millions of patients, especially in Europe, were now facing significant delays before meeting a doctor. In the US the situation was essentially the same and, like in Europe, the number of teleconsultations was rising since the beginning of the pandemic.

55-year-old Joe is aware of the current pressures on the healthcare system and he would like quick and efficient medical advice before any further intervention. Teleconsultation appeared to be the best option for Joe even if he did want a more detailed analysis of his right knee. More than a simple teleconsultation, he preferred a playful and immersive solution whilst he recovered.

After talking to his doctor who was a young and tech-savvy man Joe decided to live the experience of the virtual clinic. This meant it was possible to make a diagnostic of his knee pain by analyzing and tracking his movement in real time at home, thanks to connected devices such as gait sensors. Joe was medically monitored and then treated at home, in a virtual ward, although he would have been expedited for surgery if necessary.

A subscription to this virtual clinic was required and this could easily be reimbursed by insurance.

In order to get started Joe had to use the at home app called the "Virtual Clinic App". His phone camera had to be fixed in order to create a 3D analysis of his legs and any potential damage. All this information was duplicated and sent to his virtual hospital. But what was the point of doing it?

A real doctor involved in this virtual reality space through an avatar, interacted with Joe after receiving the personal knee imaging. Next, they had the opportunity to talk to each other as if in a medical consultation. All further interactions will take place in this virtual space the *Meta-hospital*. In this space, Joe could get treatment feedback but also workouts and entertainment service to aid his recovery. The combination of medical wellness and entertainment services encouraged Joe to recover quickly and improve his physical and mental condition. To give you a sense, Joe was able to visualize his favorite tennis court in VR and then had the opportunity to play against a great tennis player! Joe could have this great experience in a virtually realm, despite his knee problems in the real world. This is one of the playful and captivating things that the virtual world can offer. Hospital goes beyond medical treatment offering its patients different ways to be fulfilled.

In the decades to come, the virtual reality space will probably be everywhere in the area of health, even being utilized in medical operations. But don't worry; Joe won't have surgery in a virtual operating room. The only ones who will operate in a virtual operating room will be the future doctors. The metaverse will be more and more present in the Faculty of Medicine in order to offer theoretical knowledge and practical skills to the future practitioners. We will come back to that later in the "Challenges" section.

As we said, realistically a medical operation can't be completed entirely virtually! In the case of Joe, knee surgery had been planned to treat a global arthrosis causing Joe recurrent pain. The operation aimed to offer more mobility and comfort to Joe which would obviously not be possible using only a virtual solution. However, Joe was OK to share this moment online with a medical student. Joe's personal information would be inaccessible and his head blurred if desired. A virtual hospital would also be able to consider patient ethics and privacy!

A *Meta-hospital* offers endless opportunities for its patients due to the hybridization of medical and entertainment services. After having surgery, Joe could continue his rehab exercises at home by using an AR helmet to access the metaverse.

What's more, Joe's patient avatar would gather his medical history, therefore keeping an up to date medical record. He could then bring it anywhere and anytime, even to another metaverse, or to a real hospital, on condition of interoperability and reciprocity. As a unique title of property, Joe's avatar can also be monetized. In the case of Joe, his recovery time, the effect of drugs or prosthesis monitoring would all be relevant data, for not only public bodies, but the greater pharma industry and prosthetic manufacturers. This could be a new opportunity for Joe and all patients worldwide to sell totally or partially the health information related to his avatar.

At the end, this story teaches us that healthcare isn't virtual. Most of all, it is the tools and the environment around healthcare that are virtual! Joe, but also his family, will one day be confronted with digital services from an appointment booking to a teleconsultation 100% broadcasted in a metaverse. The common point between Joe, his wife and his children is what we understand what it is like to be a patient. Who has never been afraid to go to the dentist? How many children were apprehensive before their first hospital visit? Who wouldn't want to spend their stay in the hospital in a fun way? As in the case of Joe, a young child would also be more conformable exploring the virtual version of an operating room before entering a real one. Relaxing and gaming experiences through the metaverse seem interesting for the patient even if human interaction as needed.

The story of Joe is also our story whatever our age and pathology. Although the virtual hospital is a new environment, it is also a new philosophy of life.

2.2 – Build hospital & health services in the metaverse

Without a doubt the virtual reality space is large enough to build virtual hospitals and allow users to download virtual goods and services related to non-emergency medical treatment, virtual sport articles or gaming sessions. But we must remain realistic and not build castles out of air. The foundations of these systems must be solid and take into account the needs and desires of the consumer-patients. As we shall see, any type of virtual hospital and health marketplace is about concrete things such as teleconsultation, which gives patients the ability to simply talk to their doctor or get a quick and efficient diagnosis anytime and anywhere. According to Michael Kaldasch, CEO of the blockchain-based medical company *Aimedis*, healthcare based metaverse has several use cases such as therapy, consultation, educational training, research, medical training games or rehabilitation.

Definition

The concept of a virtual hospital is familiar to everyone but no one has a clear definition of it. For many years, we've heard about a virtual or digital hospital. Start-ups, big companies and governments use this term to describe telemedicine apps, connected devices and globally the modernization of the hospital.

Now let's describe what could be a virtual hospital or a virtual reality space. In a metaverse-based hospital the patient would be able to contact the right doctor, regardless of wherever they live because a virtual hospital doesn't need to have a specific location. Obviously the doctor's skills would be certified thanks to the blockchain, which will be able to prove every doctor's required certifications and past experiences. In order to access the virtual hospital, patients will have to use a headset to access a virtual or semi-virtual reality space. Another option will be to use a chat function through a virtual interface with a doctor, patients community or other type of actors. This would be popular amongst young adults as there is clear evidence that 20% of young adults opt for text messaging or chatting[2]. Pre-visits for children, teleconsultation for everyone or physical therapy for people having joints problems could be made with an AI-driven avatar or a real doctor using the metaverse. Medical operation will be excluded but depending on the severity of your symptoms we could imagine virtual emergency departments with entertaining and fanciful environment.

In the end, hospitals and services based on a metaverse will offer a range of online consultations, therapeutic exercises, fun environments and comfort for patients whilst also avoiding long waiting time. It will also be a new gateway where users will own their own health personal information through a digital title of property called an NFT.

The metaverse hospital will allow international patients to have a new experience by experiencing a broad range of services and treatments in real-time during their trip. Further, patients can also have an immersive remote consultation with healthcare providers through their avatars without leaving their homes. This also helps solve the issue of long waits and distance barriers, as patients can interact with their doctors in an immersive consultation in the virtual hospital.

Use cases & opportunities

Metaverse & Telehealth

Putting telehealth in a metaverse is maybe the most promising and well-known area investigated in virtual reality. More than just a promise, projects already exist, such as, in South Asia where hospital managers think that VR, AR and the metaverse will be a useful tool for telehealth services. These managers want to amplify

---

[2]   Data Source : oliverwyman.com, Consumer Healthcare Survey 2021.
       Adressing the Needs of Engaged Consumers

patient involvement at home by using immersive tech such as VR and AR headsets to help them to recover. The "good point" is that the Covid-2019 pandemic has accelerated the use and the adoption of telemedecine in a very short time. During the first quarter of 2020 in the US, the number of telehealth visits increased by 50%, compared with the same period in the previous years[3]. The use of digital solutions to access health care services remotely and to manage health care is fully compatible in a virtual environment. The telemedicine revolution is certainly on its way. However, is it the best model for patient, healthcare professional (HCP) and consumer? What is certain is that there is a real business model for hospital networks and clinics that could rent virtual office or 3D infrastructure at a very low cost. What's more, telemedicine and continuous access to professionals through a virtual environment offers a real continuum for monitoring a patient's health. In a virtual reality space, which is dedicated to health & wellness, the notion of care is not subject to the concept of time, location or nationality. In a 3D hospital or 3D clinic, patients will get medical advice, speak to their doctor and go through a medical procedure anytime, anywhere. Closed spaces such as prisons or retirement homes could also use VR and AR technology to enhance immersive experiences, especially when it comes to specialized medical consultation like in psychiatry. For instance, a doctor could support his patient during an immersive session where they will navigate a magical world in order to relieve their anxiety or improve their locomotion.

At the end, telehealth services in a metaverse would offer endless opportunities and a real continuum to support the user, patient and HCP. In the case of Joe, he would receive regular check-ups without even having to move. In addition thanks to an AI analysis of his medical imaging, a prediction of a risk of osteoarthritis would be made and shared with the right medical specialist in the vast space of inter-connected metaverse.

---

[3]   Trends in the Use of Telehealth During the Emergence of the Covid-19 Pandemic, US, January–March 2020

Metaverse & property

Property on personal data

Any type of personal data is valuable and even more when it comes to health personal data. To give you an example, the cost related to a hacked *Facebook* account is $74,5. Data harvested from a stolen European national ID card would be circa €1500[4]. One can only imagine how lucrative health personal health data would be for insurer, government or pharma industry. Health data provides valuable information on our body, our pathology and our mental health and that is why it is important to make sure we have total control on it.

In a metaverse based on blockchain, the user has a great chance to control their personal data by becoming the full owner of it. This is the magic of blockchain, it gives users the choice to keep their data instead of leaving them to a central authority such as a government, an administration, a hospital or a private insurance. The data would be decentralized and it would cut the middleman out of the digital transaction. Just imagine the new power of a patient who can own title of property on any type of data related to their body or their medical history. Would we be able to sell our MRI scan? Will its value be determined based on our reputation, our pathology or our popularity? Will a great actor's scan be worth more than the one of the general public? Let's see what the future brings regarding the creation of a metaverse NFT marketplace where the consumer, patient and professionals will sell and buy wellness content or medical information.

Property on lands

Over the last few years, big metaverse projects are creating great fanfare such as *Meta* from *Facebook, Decentraland, Sandbox,* as well as *Roblox.* Inspired by the world of gaming, these immersive universes are attracting a lot of players willing to travel to fantastic environments where they can fly or buy lands to start a new business in virtual real estate or virtual clothes.

---

[4]   Dark Web Price Index 2020

Today, everyone is able to purchase virtual land in different metaverses such as *Roblox* or The *Sandbox* in order to make a long-term investment or simply to feel like a homeowner. That being said, the big winners will certainly be companies such as *Nike, Addidas, Walmart, Gucci* or the french multinational *LVMH*. They create their own virtual spaces such as Nike with its Nikeland in *Roblox* metaverse. User can explore the sport field, showroom and also reproduce as real as possible movements in game thanks to its phone sensor called an accelerometer. This creates a fun activity and a real sporting competition on a digital platform. Almost every technological revolution contributes to the healthcare domain somehow.

Virtual lands are also interesting for health stakeholders. For instance, health metaverse companies could offer to hospital areas to rent or buy areas. Once the land has been purchased or leased, the hospital has the opportunity to offer to its patients virtual consultations with a specialist or medical training for students and medical staff.

At the end, it seems that big companies will probably take the lion's share for the purchase of land and the promotion of sport and wellness products and services. However, there is also a market for companies selling virtual space for hospitals, private hospital groups, health centers and eventually even retirement houses. Smaller actors in the fields of charity and wellness could also break out of the pack. Take the case of the coach who sells NFT fitness programs all across the world by using pre-bought virtual lands. We can also imagine a charitable association occupying a virtual space for promoting a cause and proposing calls for donations.

Metaverse & a new medical training experience

One of the most mentioned axes of metaverse in health is education. Through an immersive 3D environment based on VR or AR students, but also doctors and nurses could study and practice continuously. Giving 3D organ models, for example, like a heart or lung in a virtual operating room to students and surgeons would offer them higher levels of detail regarding human anatomy.

In addition, AR and VR could significantly improve doctor's performances according to different studies on orthopedic surgery[5], dentistry[6] or ophthalmology[7]. Virtual reality offers them a safe and accessible complement to their medical training outside of the operating room and without involving patients directly. Users gain unlimited access to simulations anywhere, anytime, all while diminishing risks. Once again, the metaverse is not subject to time or location.

As *Facebook* said in a video "the metaverse may be virtual but the impact will be real". Although this is true, it is only one aspect of a complex topic. The maturity of VR and AR technology will be imperative to building the most suitable metaverse-oriented medical training. Use and adoption by students, doctors and nurses will also be crucial although the younger generation of doctors will most probably be accustomed to using a VR headset.

Metaverse & Charity

One of the common points between the metaverse and philanthropy is this Utopian vision of a better world. Both concepts have much to learn from each other. Philanthropy can positively influence the metaverse by promoting the well-being of humankind. As proof, there currently exists an NFT philanthropy where different people could make a donation. In this way, a digital artist has the choice to redistribute the proceeds of his NFT artwork to help children in need or fund a pediatric hospital in Africa.

---

[5]   Laith K Hasan, Aryan Haratian, Michael Kim, Ioanna K Bolia, Alexander E Weber, Frank A Petrigliano, *Virtual Reality in Orthopedic Surgery Training, 2021*

[6]   Ta-Ko Huang a, Chi-Hsun Yang b, Yu-Hsin Hsieh c,d, Jen-Chyan Wang e,f, Chun-Cheng, *Augmented reality (AR) and virtual reality (VR) applied in dentistry*, 2018

[7]   John C Lin, Zane Yu, Ingrid U Scott, Paul B Greenberg, *Virtual reality training for cataract surgery operating performance in ophthalmology trainees*, 2022

What's more, you and I could also be potential contributors, if we decided to give money to a charity during a virtual concert or fund-raising dinner in the metaverse. In this scenario, a donor receives an NFT in return for their donation. A project to commemorate 75 years of UNICEF has planned to sell 1,000 data-driven non-fungible tokens (NFTs)[8]. Donating in this way has implications for both tax and management, as the information about the donor is stored on the blockchain. NFTs allow people to prove ownership of a digital asset and also a donation. Is it admissible to prove a donation and claim a tax-deductible donation? Can we have governance rights in the management of a charity?

Charity non-profits such as, a humanitarian organization fighting global poverty and world hunger, could then benefit from this "charitable" metaverse by creating original NFTs themselves and selling them through their own online shop accepting traditional physical money or cryptocurrencies. For instance, a children's hospital could sell its NFTs through its own dedicated shop or through a third platform like *Opensea*. Using *Opensea,* one of the largest web3 marketplaces for NFTs and crypto collectibles related to art, photography and sports, would be a good way to engage more people and raise money towards specific young adult audiences.

So, as you understand, an NFT is a fabulous entry point for any type of donor in the metaverse. Charity would now have a new promotional space and could have the opportunity to create consistent and positive earnings due to royalties for instance. The metaverse is becoming an additional leverage for non-profits as they can use it to further raise money for a cause!

---

[8]   UNICEF to launch UN's largest-ever NFT collection to mark 75th anniversary, https://www.unicef.org.uk

Challenges

There are numerous challenges related to healthcare and the metaverse. The first is about training and learning. Surgical training in the digital world has become more widely used and its future is very promising. However, one of the challenges is the development of realistic surgical interfaces and physical objects within the virtual environment. Engineers are working on realistic models of the human body, creating interface tools to view, hear, touch, feel, and manipulate these human body models thanks to haptic devices replicating a human sense of touch. These types of haptic systems are difficult to implement into surgery because of inherent restraints on cost, size, geometry, biocompatibility, and sterilization in contrast with certain consumer product such as a joystick. The realization of an immersive virtual world for medical training relies on the degree of realism and the maturity of AR and VR technologies. These are important issues for medical training and particularly surgical training. How can one learn effectively with low-precision technology when it comes to a job requiring total accuracy? How could a doctor become familiar with a body without accessing a real human body? These are serious matters when there are patients' lives on the line. The issue of real human interaction will globally influence the metaverse expansion in the health sector.

On the other hand, use and adoption of telemedicine and health related NFTs in a metaverse sounds like a challenge especially for those unprepared to use it or simply for those disinterested. Surely people who currently play, socialize and purchase sports-related NFTs in the digital world would be more inclined to use it in the future. These users are the most likely to engage in the healthcare metaverse. In this pool of adopters, they are potential patients, doctors or learners using surgical training or exploring a hospital just prior to an invasive medical procedure. The sustainability of the health metaverse will therefore depend on its community just like in the metaverse games. But is it relevant to create specific metaverse as, for example, in the healthcare industry or in the manufacturing sector? Or do we have to connect the different metaverses? In order to attract a large gaming community to other sectors perceived as less attractive or less "sexy". The choice to create a sectoral metaverse purely related to healthcare or to create an embedded metaverse into another metaverse (health metaverse into a gaming metaverse) would depend on the strategy of each operator. And whatever the strategy, the conception and the development of any metaverse should be compliant with international law and common ethical standards!

3 – The rising of Health2Earn

3.1 – « Making money by adopting a healthy lifestyle! »

Who has never had a lack of motivation to get active and to practice regular physical activity? We've all experienced such a type of demotivation by telling ourselves, "it's not a good day for me", or the "weather is rubbish", or "I'll do it another day". There are always pretexts for an exhaustible lack of desire. But this is tending to change with the revolution of connected sport over the last decades. People are increasingly using smart watches, smart heart rate belts or mobile apps to measure their physical activity and their vital signs. In the meanwhile, this is beginning to encourage more and more people to activate a self-tracking mode and share it with a community of users. We do sport to compare oneself to others and to show our performance. Seeing and being seen by our community is addictive for a lot of people. However, there are many other ways to be encouraged to pursue an active and healthy lifestyle. That's why I've decided to test health-to-earn solutions. What I call health-to-earn (health2earn) or, alternatively, earn your health is a new way to be rewarded by proving you're doing fitness, eating better, sleeping well or meditating. As a running enthusiast I wanted to convert my sports effort into money. When I said money I was referring to different type of rewards, which would be points, gift cards, cryptocurrencies like Bitcoin or also NFTs. I like this new approach especially since I have the opportunity to have control over my behavioral data by having the choice to monetize them or not. So now let's get practical!

It all started with my smart phone and a good dose of determination. I quickly realized that my smart phone has sensors, which do analyze some data concerning my movement. One of them is called an accelerometer and every smart phone in the world has this exact sensor. More specifically, the accelerometer can measure the number of steps but also the speed of them too. In the euphoria of the move-to-earn (move2earn) trend, where a user does physical activity in order to be rewarded, I decided to go for it!

 Over 3 weeks I ran every day and I was paid like a top athlete. I sometimes made $500 a day. It, however, didn't last long as the day I realized I did sport for the reward and not for myself I lost faith. The only goal I had was to make money without a sustainable philosophy. I needed something more focused on a healthy lifestyle and based on a wider variety of data such as nutrition, vital signs, mental health…

 And it is at this time that I heard about the *My-Health2Earn App*. By downloading it, I had the opportunity to choose an activity that could be tracked by phone or a connected device. I chose the first option in order to bring my phone during my running outings and be rewarded following the objectives I needed to reach. In addition to the goals set, the player's profile also counts. For instance, the expected level of physical activity of a senior with reduced mobility will not be the same as a regular young sportsman. This is a new type of personalized move-to-earn. At the same time, the app suggested a nutrition program in accordance with meals that I've scanned just before. Once again, I can earn tokens if I respect the recommended daily of intake of vitamins and minerals regard regarding my profile. Sleep is also analyzed and the app motivates its users to take care of their mental health. A gaming aspect is also offered in the metaverse to meet other people and live an immersive experience proposed by sport companies… The experience is offered both in the real world and in the virtual world.

 Like a good "student", I paid attention to my health by following programs and fun sessions given on the platform. I accumulated a lot of *MH2E* Tokens which is an opportunity to attend sport events in the metaverse or convert them into a promo code usable in a wide range of healthy partner restaurants all across the world!

 I am very motivated and working hard although I remain conscious of the difficulty of maintaining such a lifestyle for the long-term. On top of this, penalty tokens are allocated for those who don't practice during 1 month. It's a great incentive, especially if you're thinking about staying on the platform. Incentivization is a two-way street!

 In the end, I do not regret the health2earn app experience. It was very motivating! I enjoyed reaching the goals set and enjoyed being rewarded for healthy behaviors. What might seem unrealistic a decade ago is now possible. Any health-related data has a value and anyone (not only a company) can buy and trade their own data without going through intermediaries. Fitness, nutrition, mental health, love or addictions are many possible fields for the development of new projects in health2earn!

3.2 – The rising of Health2Earn

As we saw earlier, money is a good motivator for those sharing their medical and non-medical data such as fitness data. A new data economy is emerging and it is replacing centralized tech giants for the benefit of individuals who have the opportunity to own and profit from their data. Health2earn is a very beautiful illustration of data sovereignty in which individuals are taking control of their data. A multitude of applications is possible in the health2earn app although there are some challenges to keep these solutions sustainable and financially interesting for the user.

Definition

 Health2earn is a new concept allowing a user to earn virtual reward (tokens, NFTs) for any type of action related to their health. For example, the user has to prove that they walked, ate, slept, meditated or shared their patient data. How can one prove that? The answer is simple. The sensors in their phone are able to measure certain action like walking, running and cycling… Once the data related to an action is collected and stored into the blockchain it then becomes very difficult to falsify them. That's why decentralized technologies (blockchain) and sensors (accelerometer) are two interesting tools to prove that the user did perform these actions. Here are some illustrations:

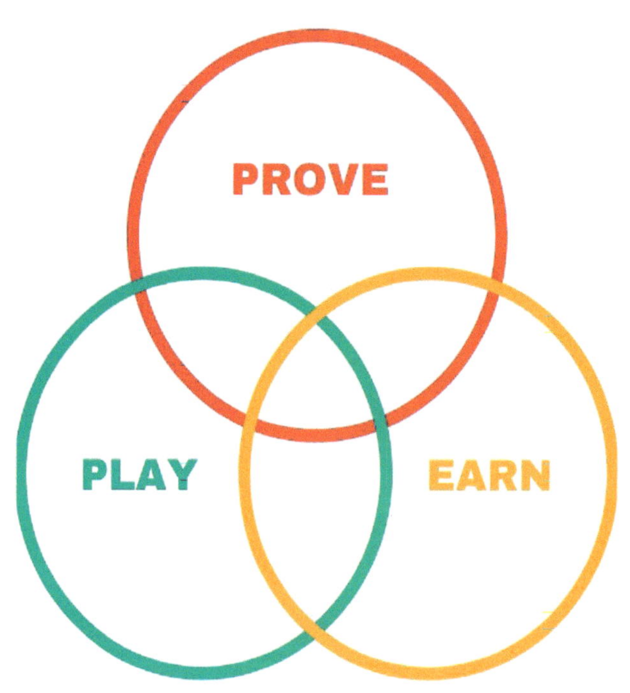

PROVE
PLAY
EARN

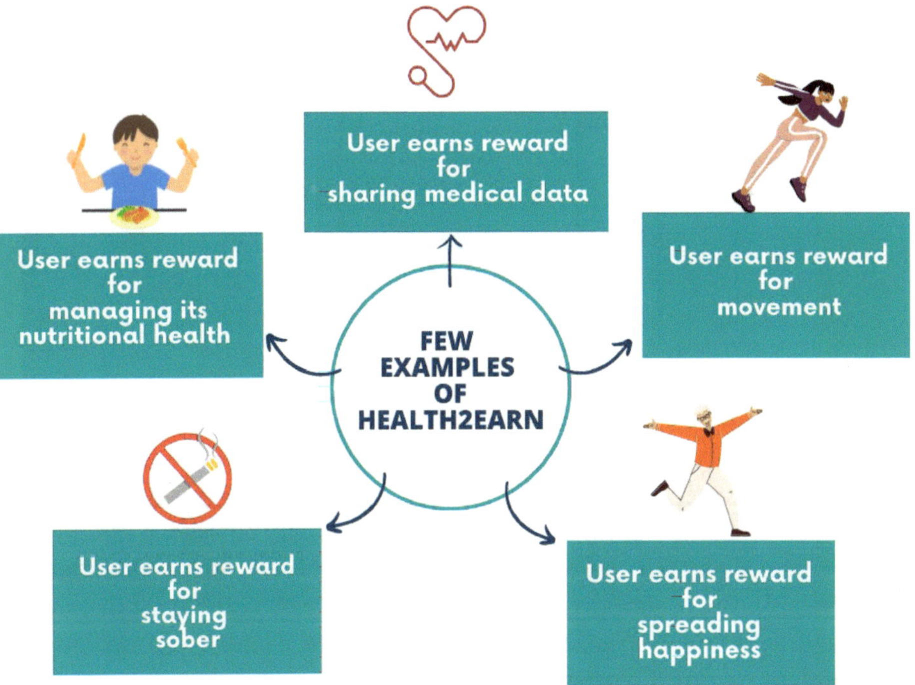

User earns reward for sharing medical data
User earns reward for managing its nutritional health
User earns reward for movement
User earns reward for staying sober
User earns reward for spreading happiness
FEW EXAMPLES OF HEALTH2EARN

Use cases & opportunities

To get active, combat sedentary behavior and obesity

 It is undeniable that health2earn promotes healthy behaviors and a way to control health data. There are clear benefits both for users and society particularly in the case of public health. In fact, the economy of the movement commonly known as "move-to-earn" could be of significant public health relevance. This concept has the potential to be a game-changer by fighting health problems like obesity. We do not claim that we will totally eradicate sedentary lifestyles or obesity thanks to the blockchain and its health-related solutions based on financial incentives. Nevertheless, according to major studies such as one in the Lancet Global Health[9], insufficient physical activity is a leading risk factor for non-communicable diseases and has a negative effect on mental health and quality of life. Sedentary lifestyles are a real problem even for those who regularly practice a sport. We are seen as sedentary if we sit or lie for more than seven hours in a day. So I can sit 7 hours a day and do 4 hours of sports a week and yet still be classed as sedentary. Therefore, it is important to get active and combat sedentary behavior, which increases the risk of obesity, cancer, osteoporosis and depression. Financial incentives seem a good motivator to increase exercise adherence in adults in the short term (<6 months) according to a meta-analysis that combines and synthesizes multiple studies. We have to be realistic. The link between regular physical activity and sedentary is complex and health2earn is a tool more than a solution. The best health2earn project will be one that will both increase the level of physical activity and reduce sedentary lifestyles. Strategic partnership with a public health

---

9 Regina Guthold, Gretchen A Stevens, Leanne M Riley, Fiona C Bull, *Worldwide trends in insufficient physical activity from 2001 to 2016: a pooled analysis of 358 population-based surveys with 1·9 million participants*, 2018

system will also be crucial for start-ups and companies working in this field. Displaying exactly this, *Sweatcoin* has launched a Diabetes Prevention partnership with the National Health Service (NHS) in South West London. It's a win-win model. The NHS benefits from a mobile app that promotes physical activity, which in turn will reduce obesity and its huge associated public costs. Additionally, *Sweatcoin* can acquire a large number of users by promoting and incentivising physical activity among the English population.

To promote mental health through incentives & community

We live in a fast-moving society where everything can seem like a whirlwind! News, tech, work, leisure... everything is happening! Since the beginning of the COVID-19 pandemic a global crisis for health has emerged fueling short and long-term stresses and undermining the mental health of millions of people across the globe according to the world health organization (WHO). Mental health is one thing, and happiness is another. Mental health is defined as an integral part of our general health and well-being and is a basic human right as defined by the WHO. Happiness is a concept that is still being debated. According to American psychiatrist and geneticist, Claude Robert Cloninger, happiness can be described as the state of well-being that is often characterized by positive emotions ranging from contentment to intense joy. Is the pursuit of happiness an illusion? Can we guarantee happiness and avoid mental health disorders? As crazy as it seems, using the metaverse and giving financial incentives could be useful in promoting mental health and happiness.

We know that navigating and receiving positive stimuli combined with health knowledge could be a valuable tool for public health and mental health[10]. Many entrepreneurs and start-ups are entering

---

[10] Shaun W Jerdan , Mark Grindle , Hugo C van Woerden , Maged N Kamel Boulos, *Head-Mounted Virtual Reality and Mental Health: Critical Review of Current Research*, 2018

the metaverse market by offering VR programs for depressed people, seniors and young people with cognitive impairment. The metaverse is an interesting place to medically treat this type of person, especially younger populations, such as teenagers and young adults, who are often familiar with the digital world. The metaverse is maybe the solution but it could also be the problem! Spending too much time in a digital environment can negatively impact our ability to engage in real life. Social networks and the gaming universe are the perfect example. Like anything, balance is key! What's more, the metaverse and NFTs also have an ethical dimension. NFT projects like *AussieMates* NFT can play an important role in promoting better mental health and physical well-being through offering a supportive community. The team wants to develop a Mental Health Metaverse Hub. The concept of community will be crucial, regardless of whether it is real or virtual. The Mental Health Hub will let people talk, tackle mental health stigma and will encourage them to live normally. People but also founders have a role to play in this fight. Community incentives could reward token or NFT holders for promoting mental health, well-being focused in-real life and happiness as discussed below.

To promote happiness through incentive & community

For the Dalai Lama "the very purpose of life is to seek happiness." Feeling positive more than negative is maybe the most characteristic feature of happiness. Happiness is more a matter of global satisfaction than money. However, money certainly does contribute to this state of satisfaction. Money brings serenity and safety for not only ourselves, but also for our family, friends and charity organizations. It is not inconsistent to imagine a sort of "happiness tokenization" where you are rewarded to spread joy! Rewarding someone by allocating a token is not a bad idea to motivate others to spread happiness. Of course, this implies that happiness can be measured. Community and network are a driving force for change and good. No matter the size, the community, whether it is real or virtual, must be interactive. Founders and users have to be involved from the beginning of the project by sharing their insights and spreading joy and optimism in the social network. A new type of happiness-to-earn could emerge by allocating a token in return for a good deed, like funding mental health programs for example. A person could be rewarded after proving their happiness or by making other people happy. This would be symbolic and financial reward work.

For employers and their employee

Health2earn is very powerful to engage employees in a comprehensive health program that makes a real difference in their lives. Such programs may include workouts, nutrition advice or posture exercises for office workers. In this case, a decentralized solution such as a mobile app helps employees keep track of their health behavior. The decentralized app called Dapp associated to fitness tracker or VR tools is generally connected to an existing company willing to offer health programs to interested employees. Through these programs, companies have access to some personal data like heart rate, steps, localization, blood pressure… Then, workers who have completed their health goals are rewarded by their employer with gifts such as a gym pass or travel coupons. It is a win-win, between a company looking for healthy employees who are less inclined to be absent due to sickness, and for the employee who will reduce the chances of developing medical problems later in life (depression, cardiovascular diseases, cancer and diabetes). What is the benefit for companies? Companies would benefit from reduced health costs regarding employer-provided coverage and wellness programs that are currently offered by the company. These are stated to be two times more expensive than move-to-earn solutions according to the estimation of certain fitness-finance start-ups.

For insurance companies

For many years, insurance companies have been interested in the lifestyle of their members. Personal data has been the new gold for a few decades. Health and life insurance companies have understood the value of this health gold. Creating a virtual community of insured members who are involved in a health2earn program is a potential strategic investment. Although the consent of insured people must be required before enrolling them in a health2earn program, it is really worthwhile to make the user active and not passive as we see in the current insurance model. This issue is all the more sensitive when it comes to data related to the health of a user. Indeed, health personal data is sensitive and its use for different purposes will be contrary to the general data protection regulation (GDPR) in force in Europe. After receiving a user's consent, incentives for physical activities could be allocated to them. The insurer will reward their member for completing health goals. This can also be seen as a win-win situation as in the previous model. The insurance company can extract real-time data through a partner Dapp or through an in-house solution in order to predict long-term disease or accident risk and re-evaluate their rate almost instantly. To protect the consumer, one could imagine that insurance rate adjustment would only be upward as a reward and not act as a penalty.

Challenges

Health2earn opportunities seem promising even if a few obstacles might hinder its progress. Most of the current move-to-earn requires the user to invest. However, Oleg Fomenko, co-founder of *Sweatcoin* points out that move2earn solutions should be separated from projects that are pay-to-play and are charging for the right to participate. Requiring a fee makes their potential markets tiny and their business model unsustainable. For instance, in certain games, you have to buy a digital sneaker (which is an NFT) before playing the game. The price can reach up to $2,000 for just one digital item! The cost of a virtual shoe is clearly a problem often related to the price of the required cryptocurrency. There is a double danger. The user may see the price of the same shoe at half the price, which could be considered as a financial loss. The project leader takes the risk of discouraging potential user. Over time, this situation will negatively impact the community and, ultimately, the whole project.

The second problem, which is related to the first, is that repeated and excessive investments in an NFT, such as digital running shoes or an avatar, generates more losses than revenue. This is not an incentive program for a user.

Now let's talk about the purpose of these games. The psychological aspect of health2earn is a double-edged sword. Being competitive is good and useful for achieving one's goals, preserving one's health and making more money. However, many users just play to make money without worrying about the health and well-being aspect. Some people play for fun, other play for making money.

The last point is about use and adoption of health2earn. As we've seen, user involvement and the weight of the community are crucial for the sustain sustainability of the project. Use and adoption of a health2earn program requires some equipment. In different cases, you have to use a smartphone, maybe some trackers, a VR headset and a wallet in order to receive and store your reward in the form of digital currency. But who has ever created a health2earn wallet? Who knows how to convert their cryptocurrency into a coupon, which can be used in real life? All these questions define the new decentralized economy in which health2earn exists within. The success of this economy will depend on usage and acceptance by non-tech people. We are just at the beginning of the health2earn adoption lifestyle!

4 – The metaverse & the life sciences industry

4.1 – Welcome to a meta-pharmacy!

The metaverse is about having an immersive experience. In the future, people will have the opportunity to buy drugs and medical devices in different metaverse. Even more the prescription will be able to be obtained in these virtual worlds! Without leaving home, by using a VR headset or connected contact lenses, I'm able to access a lot of pharmacies and find many offers to participate in paid clinical research trials. During my virtual exploration, a giant digital billboard continuously displays the following message: "Earn up to $10,000!" It is very attractive and I wonder what to do. Is it a real or digital trial? Will it be safe? I'm a little confused even if it is pretty lucrative! Anyway, I continue my exploration into finding a pharmacy in the metaverse. After some research, I have found the right virtual pharmacy. It is located in my favorite metaverse called *"FunCity"*. And by the way, I saw a few people from my community visiting the same virtual pharmacy. Interaction and fun experience within the community makes it more attractive and it's what I like.

Entering a drugstore is not very difficult in a metaverse. A lot of products are for sale such as candy, gums, syrup, luxury fragrance but also probiotics to improve gut health. The choice is wide and the products are varied. All of these products are shown in their digitalized version and some of them are NFTs. For instance, 1000 pieces of the latest fragrance have been sold recently. The most expensive piece from the collection, *"In the air"*, by a famous Japanese artist sold for $1,500! The level of realism and 3D visual effects are absolutely amazing. Even if all of that seems simple, I have to verify my account with a valid ID whether to buy drugs or a simple syrup. Once my identity has been validated, I can order fragrance, drugs or any type of product offered in this virtual drugstore. When my ID is verified, it analyzes all the medical information related to myself, including my medical history and medical prescriptions. If I don't have a prescription for a specific drug, the transaction cannot be made. Once I have filled my virtual cart, I choose to pay in *Healthy Super Coin* (MSC) which is a worldwide decentralized currency accepted by drugstores, sports coaches, healers and sports companies… The 3D experience was fun and I just got a notification telling me that my package will arrive within 3-7 days. In the meanwhile and to thank me for my loyalty, I receive a free code for a nutrition consultation, which is valid for the next 6 months. Once the code is used for that first appointment, I should be able to log into the designated pharmacy to meet a nutritionist in a 3D space. The consultation will be in a virtual private room (Room 3) and elements will appear during the session, such as virtual ailments, which I can eat in order to analyze eating behavior and the effects on my body.

At home, the experience continues beyond this 100% virtual world with mixed reality, which is a sort of virtual continuum in the real life. The interaction seems more intuitive and allows me to visualize in 3D the drug I ordered. I have access to a lot of information. For example, I have an instant and permanent access to the doctor's instructions even if I forget them. The 3D image of the medication, that I have in front of me in my living room is also a useful AR tool to get alerts when my medication is going to expire or even just to remind me to take the medicine.

Only five days later, my package has arrived. The order is complete and undamaged. And as a bonus, I find inside the package a QR code to access a metaverse entertainment where I can attend different virtual concerts. I have full access to this immersive experience for a month, and that's exciting because at one of my favorite pop singers will be performing!

4.2 – A new playground for the life sciences industry?

Definition

There is currently no definition of what constitutes a "pharmaverse" or a metaverse related to the life sciences industry! On the 28th of February 2022, *CVS Health* which is an American retail pharmacy and health care company has filled a patent in order to provide, in the near future, "downloadable virtual goods, consumer goods, prescription drugs, health, wellness, beauty, personal care products and general merchandise" according to the United States Patent and Trademark Office. It also referred to digital assets and digital collectibles sold as non-fungible token (NFTs). However, it is too soon to assess how the industry will respond. The life sciences industry is a large industry with a lot of players, including companies operating in the field of research, pharmaceuticals, biotechnology, cosmetics, medical devices and solutions offering benefits to human health. Every sector has its own specific needs and will develop new virtual forms of relationships with their individual consumers.

Use cases & opportunities

A new relationship between pharmacists and customers

The pharmacist-patient relationship is crucial in order to promote patient engagement. A strong relationship between the two parties can lead to better patient satisfaction and can benefit the therapy's success. Human factors play a decisive role in ensuring a good relationship based on communication and goodwill. Besides this major factor, efficiency in drug delivery is a key point to explore. That's why pharmacies have an interest to offer their goods and services in the existing metaverse or in their own metaverse. As we've seen in *"FunCity"*, there's no need to go to a physical pharmacy to get drugs, quasi-drugs or gums! When the products are available and ready, it get's processed in a pharmacy. Metaverse facilitates drug delivery and creates a sort of continuity between a pharmacy and a home. The metaverse is progressively blurring the lines between the physical and the virtual world. The longer-term impact will change the fundamentals of pharmacist-patient relationships. The communication between the pharmacist and their patients will be the same but it will be more digital than real. This gain in time regarding logistics and drug management for the pharmacist will allow pharmacists to schedule more digital sessions in a 3D space than in a physical pharmacy. It is also very likely that the service rendered to the patient will be more personalized. Metaverse will be an important milestone for pharmacies!

A new business model for pharmacies

 As many know, a pharmacies business model is based on selling over-the-counter drugs, prescription drugs, medical equipment and health and beauty products. Due to strict legal regulations in many countries, the sector, fortunately, doesn't sell as much as e-commerce retail in the fashion industry. However, since the beginning of the Covid-19 pandemic, many processes have been digitized and online services continue to grow. In parallel, the metaverse is becoming the next big social networking space, which is a boon for pharmacies and their online services. In the next decades, pharmacies should be able to put the necessary mechanisms to offer an online shopping experience by using VR. New types of 3D counseling sessions in the fields of nutritional advice, pre-pregnancy counseling and quitting smoking will be provided using various technologies. The metaverse is a virgin land for pharmacies and other drugstores. The possibilities are endless especially in terms of advertising. Pharmacies and drugstores will strengthen their virtual presence by purchasing territories and by forming partnerships with lots of virtual spaces, products and services. The most successful marketing and advertising campaigns will surely depend on national regulation. For instance, in the US, there are essentially no regulations for advertising over-the-counter (OTC) drugs. Just prescription drugs, and certain kinds of medical devices like hearing aids, are regulated by the FDA. In Europe, mistrust is common, particularly among European citizens, and doctors regarding advertising for prescription drugs. National law will have an impact on drug and health product ads in the metaverse. But that being said, services offered by pharmacies and drugstores are now much less regulated, or entirely deregulated which is an excellent opportunity for these virtual actors.

New horizons for the pharmaceutical companies & patient communities

The Covid-19 pandemic has changed our patient and consumer uses. How many times have we seen the number of steps we took thanks to our smartwatch? Who has thought of not contacting a doctor for a consultation due to lockdowns? Digital health monitoring and wearable technology are gradually becoming the norm and the pharmaceutical sector has understood this well. The start of the pandemic has accelerated the transition from on-site clinical trial monitoring to remote monitoring providing an access to real-time data from anywhere.

Pharmaceutical companies have the opportunity to complete clinical trials at lower costs by collecting a lot of personal data quickly. The more people who share their data in the metaverse, the easier it will be to run clinical trials at scale. The metaverse offers pharmaceutical companies a new way of recruiting subjects who have the appropriate age, gender or diseases required for the study. This could save a lot of time, especially when we consider that the average recruitment time for drug development is normally around 5 months. The metaverse is a pool of potential participants for clinical trials. If the number of participants is not enough in the metaverse, the use of twin technology seems relevant to run clinical trials. In a metaverse, a digital twin is a virtual model representing a human being, a product or a process. In a clinical trial, a digital twin could exist in the form of a human and all its attributes such as organs, tissues, DNA and so on. Thanks to VR technology, the investigator and researchers would be able to visualize in 3D the progression of cancer on certain organs and cells. The pharmaceutical industry will also be able to test new processes more easily thereby improving their processes and their training. They could also present their latest drugs during an international, giant virtual event inviting doctors from all around the world. From the trial to the promotion, the experience will be more immersive, user-friendly and adjusted to the needs of the patient, researchers, HCP and all the people working in this sector. Let's not forget start-ups that have the opportunity to play their cards right when they meet the need of a pharmaceutical industry. Therefore, it will not be surprising that companies working on move2earn are part of a clinical trial where the study of a drug is combined with physical activity.

Metaverse will be the place where science, tech, creativity and patient communities come together to share ideas and invent new ways to experience engagement.

Challenges

The metaverse is a new tool for life science companies that are designing and promoting a drug. For patients it is a useful gateway to learn more about treatments and also eventually pay for it. However, this new experience has limits regarding legal and regulatory challenges. Added to these limitations is the extent of on-line promotion and sales. Will pharmaceutical companies, drugstores and pharmacies communicate digitally on their products (drug, quasi-drugs…) or on their services (nutrition counseling, test…)? Will the sales for prescription drugs be prohibited in the metaverse due to national regulation or ethical reasons? Nothing is certain, but the legal privacy framework in the US or Europe will continue to promote and protect human rights through both the GDPR in the European Union and the Health Insurance Portability and Accountability Ac in the US. The concept of consent is central in both regulations. The metaverse should take into account what will be possible and what will not be permitted in the 3D space. As a first step, we could imagine a virtual world where a lot of non-medical products and wellness services are marketed first. It could be online relaxing sessions for patients or healthy cooking workshops for 10 adults in the 3D space. These offerings are not sensitive regarding personal health data and they could operate in a flexible legal framework. However, any type of service requiring patient consent for medical purpose will require special attention by developers in terms of regulation and ethics. The last challenge for private and public companies looking to increase their footprint in the metaverse will be whether or not they use another metaverse to develop their activity. Will they integrate into another metaverse or will they create their own metaverse? For time and technical reasons, a large part of these projects will use existing metaverse and will exploit the fact that metaverse will be more and more interoperable to connect multiple metaverse to each other. Right now, it is unclear whether leading companies in the healthcare industry such as *CVS Health* will market their products and services on an existing metaverse platform or if they will need to create a proprietary version from scratch.

 In time, the life science industry needs much more education to understand and develop their presence in the metaverse. For now, these companies need external developers because they don't have a video game or programming culture according to the experts I interrogated. This industry has a lot of money, especially when considering the world's 10 biggest pharmaceutical companies. However, a large part of their team doesn't realize the virtual opportunities available to them. They probably need new blood to bring this subject to the oldest employees!

5 – Metaverse for vulnerable populations (seniors, disabled people...)

5.1 - The Story of "Abuelita"

Maria Teresa called "Abuelita" by her children and grandchildren is a loving grandmother. Now 75 years old, Abuelita continues to live well even if she has been diagnosed with Parkinson's disease a couple of years ago. She remembers the day she was diagnosed with Parkinson symptoms. It all started with a persistent pain in her right arm. After consulting a doctor, she eventually had an answer. The diagnosis revealed a long-term degenerative disorder commonly known as Parkinson's. In the moment, it was so raw for Abuelita and her family. She thought it was merely a small injury but it was, in fact, early symptoms of Parkinson's diseases. Over the years, Abuelita and her family got used to living life "more slowly". She regularly has tremors and finds it difficult to move and keep her balance.

Being an optimist, she tried some experimental rehabilitation such as one using an automatic virtual environment using treadmills and strength training. The results were incredible! Through this immersive experience, Abuelita improved her balance. She has much more energy and her muscle reactivity is better. However, this semi-virtual environment is quite expensive and requires a lot of organization.

In the meanwhile, Abuelita is happy. Since the diagnosis, she has already visited many countries such as Korea, Japan, Australia and France. She's now learning Argentine tango and she takes cooking lessons once a week! Social interactions are very important for her. However, the disease progresses year after year. Drug treatments and surgery are possible but she doesn't want to hear, or consider, these options. She is looking for an alternative to compensate for the signs and symptoms she feels. Indeed, Parkinson's disease negatively impacts her everyday life. She has to reduce physical activity and she has sleep disorders. In addition, she feels a certain stiffness and a slowing of her movements. Her past experience using a treadmill in a semi-virtual environment was fruitful but not 100% immersive like in an online metaverse. Since then, the development of haptic technologies have grown much more accurate and realistic. The mere use of a wearable haptic provides good sensations when you touch something in a virtual space. Feeling cold or feeling hot is now possible thanks to a haptic suit or haptic gloves, whereby you can be in real-feel contact with a virtual space replicating a desert or a mountain. You can feel this sensation as if you were actually there. Abuelita is optimistic and she believes technology is a tremendous enabler. So, she decides to test haptic gloves and a VR headset to head into a virtual world.

 The first steps are strange but it is easy enough to get used to. This entire virtual space is much larger than the semi-virtual environment she experimented before, which didn't have a VR headset. The sensations are tenfold by using haptic suits including gloves, kneepads and wearable haptic ankles. More than a gadget, the wearable haptic ankles have a real purpose for improving the gait in Parkinson's patients. Abuelita loves the many long walks along the virtual seafront through which she can access from her favorite metaverse called *Sun & Relaxing City*. During this immersive experience, Abuelita's gait ability becomes more fluid due to the processing of haptic stimuli. Haptic technology allows her to perceive the virtual world with a new sensorial dimension. Better yet, the feel of the sea breeze and the social interaction with her two grandchildren using the same metaverse are ultra realistic. Her two grandchildren Julia and Markus who live respectively in New York and Paris are regularly joining their grandma in *Sun & Relaxing City* to walk around the city and have a chat with her. It is also very pleasant for her to hold their hands virtually with an incredible sense of touch even if they live far away. Haptic tech is stimulating the feeling of touch in the virtual interaction. For the first time since she was diagnosed with Parkinson's, she no longer feels tremors and muscle rigidity during an immersive session. Each time she navigates the virtual world, Abuelita start to lose feeling in parts of her body. It is a kind of disincarnation, or disembodiment, where the relation to the sick body doesn't exist anymore. Reality no longer opposes the virtual. Reality is now the virtual!

5.2 – It's time to build a better Metaverse! Is a responsible & inclusive metaverse a utopia?

Definition

The concept of good and evil is a dichotomy that had been used for a very long time. The notion of 'good' is defined by some as something useful. It was for example, the definition of the philosopher Baruch Spinoza. What is good could help every single group including the most vulnerable. A concern for others and a belief in fairness encourages us all to think about what can be done to protect the vulnerable and minority populations. That's why I call for the introduction of an unlimited liability from the design and the conception of the metaverse project. This is even more important when it comes to disability or ageing. In the same way, European regulation requires organizations to adopt the principles of "privacy by design and by default". We must set ethical standards to respond to human vulnerability. In this sense, we share some use cases and opportunities to preserve the body and mind of most vulnerable people through the digital space.

Use cases & opportunities

Metaverse for functional autonomy

In the virtual world the concept of gravity doesn't exist anymore which could be promising for people who have suffered damage to the central nervous system through stroke, myopathy or trauma after a car accident. VR could be an interesting tool to stimulate brain plasticity and motor learning for this range of patients. What a pleasure to imagine a hemiplagic patient after a stroke doing rehab while feeling his body floating in 3D space. The development of rehab metaverse is just beginning but its potential is huge to aid patients to relearn every day activities such as eating, bathing and any type of functional mobility. In other words, the metaverse could be a place where disabled people can be independent.

For rehab & social inclusion

As said before, VR is a promising technological tool to ensure the inclusion of people with disabilities. For instance, big companies such as *Samsung* or *Microsoft* have developed VR programs for different types of blind people. They offer technological assistance in order to adjust vision or help children understand social interaction despite their disability. In addition to these big public products & services, a few organizations and hospitals moved into the field of metaverse to create new opportunities for patients. The World Federation for Neuro Rehabilitation (WFNR) and some hospitals have already secured their space in the *Aimedis* Health City Metaverse according to its CEO, Michael Kaldasch. Ultimately, *Aimedis* tends to be a virtual gateway for hospitals, clinics, universities, insurance companies, pharmacies and any type of healthcare related entities. As stated by Michael Kaldasch, all the developments were made for patient that's why they've built patient community in neuro-rehab. What's more, neuro-rehab seems to be one the most relevant field in the metaverse enabling users to connect, interact, rehabilitate and receive online treatment in a 3D space. Neuro-rehab is a global medical process offering physical, sensorial, cognitive, psychological and social therapies to maximize the chances of patient recovery. So the virtual world seems to be a place where researchers and developers could create innovative approaches to increase a patients' gait and balance during the recovery phase as some research has shown. The creation of move2earn apps is an interesting idea where more work could be done in order to offer new challenges for the user. We could imagine new business models that reward patients for their engagement. In the meantime, we must not forget learning in medicine and neurosciences, which might be proposed in a metaverse game for instance. Autonomy is a sector involving lots of people such as patients in rehab and parts of the population who are losing their autonomy due to aging and persistent mental disorders.

For ageing

 An ageing population has been a growing demographic group in society for many years. This phenomenon will be more pronounced in young populations like in Africa. This aged population will reach 1.5 billion by 2050 according to the United Nations (UN)[11]. A loss of autonomy among the aged is correlated to that fact, even if certain elements are difficult to predict. But, in any case, factors influencing healthy ageing are known. The functional limitations of the older adult appear with age (physical, sensory impairments and cognitive disabilities). These diseases and functional limitations are potentially sources of disability and loss of autonomy. This is where the metaverse can come into play! Virtual reality has already proved its worth in various "serious games" for cognitive stimulation in people with Alzheimer's or Parkinson's disease. Virtual reality allows these users to reduce the impact of the neurological diseases. Same for functional, postural rehabilitation or any type of games offered in 3D spaces, for example, imagine a virtual home where the elderly can fully perceive their environment yet cannot fall in real life.

The metaverse might be the next step in extended reality including VR, AR and mixed reality. It will offer senior populations but also

---

[11]   World Population Ageing 2019 Report - United Nations

to patients a hybrid experience with an emphasis on social and content dimensions. A strong data model with best practices and a high level of data privacy will be necessary for collecting real-time data on movement and gait of older people. The use of a digital twin could be interesting to make the link between the real world and the digital world. Metaverse is undoubtedly promising for those who are maturing with age! However, research is needed to define the impact of the metaverse on ageing gracefully in the long term.

Metaverse for social relations

We are social beings with an appetite to communicate and build friendships and love relationships. Social relationships define an essential aspect of our social being. Building a sustainable metaverse without connecting people is like building strong relationships without meeting any people! *Facebook* and other big social networks have become, over the years, a social fact because they allow their users to share messages, pictures and any type of personal or impersonal information. The reason for their success is surely "social interaction". But as we will see in the "Challenges" section, this sociability can also be very isolating. To be successful and sustainable, the metaverse must leave a positive impact on their users, especially those from vulnerable communities. And so, it's a paradox! The search for individual interest is also crucial in terms of use and adoption. In general, many factors come into play such as economic, social and cultural factors. These factors determine the way the average user engages with social networks. Regarding vulnerable populations, such as the older generation or disabled people, age-related factors and the appropriation of technology must not be disregarded. How does a senior who has never paid in cryptocurrency purchase an item in the metaverse? Is it easy for a disabled person with gripping difficulties to wear a VR headset? Will an autistic person be able to communicate through an avatar even if this person has difficulty understanding humor and figurative speech in the real world? The metaverse is probably an opportunity to reach young and tech-savvy consumers but no one knows if it will be able to reach disabled people or the older population. In the following section you will be introduced to some metaverse applications which could be developed specifically for vulnerable people.

To reduce social isolation by creating a community

According to the WHO and the UN, social isolation and loneliness are widespread among older people in some countries and regions including the USA, China, Europe and Latin America. These problems are not limited to social interactions. The risks of social isolation and loneliness are massive as they have consequences on human life expectancy by impacting a person's mental and physical health. These risks could be mitigated by the possibilities offered by a virtual community in the metaverse. We could imagine virtual age-friendly communities with an access from nursing homes, senior service residences or even from at home. A nurse, a member of their family or a volunteer, could assist the elderly person in understanding and using the technological tools. Strategies are necessary to build physical and virtual communities and they have the potential to help reduce social isolation as many research projects have shown in the past. However, an appropriate and accessible technology is crucial to keep seniors and globally vulnerable people connected.

A win-win model for seniors and sociomedical stakeholders

By building virtual ancillary products and services on the metaverse, organizations such as nursing homes, associations or city departments for the aging have an opportunity to create several gateways for senior citizen. Following this logic, the most important Swiss organization offering information and services for seniors bought virtual lands on *The Sandbox* and *Decentraland* for 15,000 Swiss Francs. The purpose of its purchase is to offer a digital course center or counseling center in the metaverse according to *Pro Senectute* Both Basels. The stakes are high, mostly linked to the changing ways of interacting and being part of a community. On the other hand, the organization is duplicating its services in the virtual world to communicate and reinforce its presence among current and future seniors generation. It is a bet on the future!

To offer an immersive experience for people suffering from a memory disorder

It seems that social interaction can reduce certain type of neurodegenerative diseases like Alzheimer. This is the result of a study conducted with 10,228 participants. The questionnaire investigated their social contacts and asked about relationships with relatives and friends living outside of their household. After investigating, researchers found that more frequent social contact with friends at age 60 correlated with a lower dementia risk. More specifically, social activity in a persons 60s may lower dementia risk by 12%![12] No matter what anyone says, sociability could be crucial in preventing dementia. After the occurrence of the disease, the metaverse is also able to play a role in supporting people willing to find memories of their past and improve communication with family and caregivers. What we call "immersive reminiscence" could help an old senior suffering from memory disorder. By using the metaverse and its related tools, people with dementia or an amnesiac could relive again a pleasant time spent in their family home or experience an unforgettable summer by the sea. The power of emotions arising from the reminiscence experience will make using the metaverse successful.

Fight against social exclusion by introducing poverty in the metaverse!

In March 2022, a French non-profit organization called *Entourage* introduced the first virtual homeless avatar in the metaverse to raise awareness about the risk of exclusion inherent in the 3D space. According to the association, more and more people are ultra-connected and this will continue into the metaverse. But at the same

---

[12] Sommerlad A, Sabia S, Singh-Manoux A, Lewis G, Livingston G, *Association of social contact with dementia and cognition: 28-year follow-up of the Whitehall II cohort study*, 2019

time, people are increasingly isolated in front of screens. There is an imbalance between social interaction in the real life and relationships in the virtual world. The message is therefore political and philosophical. Policy makers and tech entrepreneurs have a real responsibility to preserve social interaction in both worlds. This virtual homeless person named Will is now a symbol illustrating a common isolation in big cities, where people's connections with homeless people are often impersonal. Will is an ambassador for excluded people who live in the real world but also for those who will interact in the metaverse. In a metaverse where a Gucci bag is sold for over $4,000, the risk of exclusion is well present. Similar social inequalities that occured previously in the real world might be repeated in the metaverse. But, even if the inequalities are inexorably reproduced and repeated, the metaverse offers some immersive services and tools to make medical, social or charitable projects prosper. Will's biggest challenge is also to bring a positive energy to build a responsible & inclusive metaverse that will not simply be a utopia!

Challenges

The biggest challenge for motivating vulnerable populations to enter the metaverse is inclusion! Inclusion can be a short or long process where developers and vulnerable people learn from each other to create the best possible experience. It is necessary to include future users in the design work from the beginning, so that the product can meet the users desires and needs. This will also avoid any technological and social divide. Developers, tech project managers and public bodies have to keep in mind that the technological gap is often due to social divisions. That's why a diverse range of people including the elderly, disabled people and minorities should be included in the project's design and development. Inclusion is also about learning and teaching.

We have to know what vulnerable users want in terms of user experience (UX) or the price they could reasonably afford. For instance, one of the most advanced haptic gloves currently costs about $4,500 which is not accessible for a lot of people across the world. So, when can this technology become mainstream? When will haptic gloves become more affordable for everyone? In a world where approximately 80% of older people by 2050 will be living in low and middle-income countries, the question of inclusion through age-inclusive technology adoption is also critical for the future of functional and social autonomy. In my opinion, the purchase price will remain very high as significant investment in terms of research and development is required at the outset. However, it could become accessible tech for everyone thanks to the location-based entertainment model, which would allow consumers to live fun and amazing experiences through virtual reality at a lower cost. This haptic technology that offers a high level of sensitivity whilst in the virtual experience could be a benefit for patients in rehab but also for everyone willing to understand patient pain and difficulties. For instance, a hospital in Belgium has invited caregivers and family to experience what a patient with multiple sclerosis (MS) feels. They have used haptic gloves associated with a helmet to perceive MS symptoms like tremors and restriction of movement. Once again virtual reality tools are an advocacy tool to raise awareness about frailty and vulnerability. The virtual world can be, and should be, for vulnerable users and for the people surrounding him.

To conclude, the risk of isolation and dependence related to the digital world also affects vulnerable people. The metaverse connects people whilst simultaneously isolating them, therefore being a paradoxical notion. That's why, the design and development of the metaverse for this kind of population will need to be carefully examined. For instance, the metaverse should not isolate seniors and people with neurological disorders. They need an anchor to reality to preserve their balance between the two worlds. Let's make immersive session for the elderly and vulnerable people by putting them in a group and letting them feel the same sensation at the same time. Social cohesion is not a luxury but a necessity especially when it comes to vulnerable people. There are still so many philosophical and ethical issues to take into consideration for this population but also for the general population. Introducing ethics into the digital world is essential!

AFTERWORD

An unexpected result of writing a book about metaverse is that I spent more time in the real world than the digital world! Even if there is hybridization between our human society and virtual communities, especially in the gaming area, we can legitimately say the metaverse is no longer science fiction. It tends to offer us an alternative universe in the digital world, one where we can live and be treated medically as needed! More than a fiction, Melinda, Joe and Abuelita are among us. The technology is already here and I hope citizens will take advantage of this opportunity.

 The digital world is a real serious track for the health and well-being sector regarding the diversity of stakeholders interested in it. From hospitals to sporting goods manufacturers, they all want a place in the metaverse. The reasons are money and time! The metaverse could save time and money by ensuring the highest quality of hospital care at a lower cost, generating additional revenues for a private actor or diminishing travel cost where physical presence is not really required. In other words, metaverse is a world of optimization where people and companies are interconnected in 3D spaces. It's a new world of experiences offering new inclusive ways of interacting in spaces shaped by human beings for human beings. Why do I say that? Why insist on the human being? Like AI, the metaverse doesn't have a full existence because both were created by humans. Every emotion, representation and concrete thing that is transposed into the metaverse come from real life. It comes from humans and more precisely the human unconscious, which generates our feelings, emotions and representations. It is also interesting to see many types of metaverse. Those that are permanent and those that are temporary. Some that offer psychedelic experiences in an imaginary environment that are very colorful like a cartoon. Others offer human centered experiences by reproducing a real human face in a life-like virtual landscape. In my opinion, these types of universes are relevant especially if they are suitable for a specific audience. I have had many conversations with many of the big players in metaverse related to healthcare and other matters. Some believe that when it comes to a patient or vulnerable person metaverse has to be human-centric while some think that a cartoon-like environment could be interesting for pediatric patients. But, in any case, AI and metaverse are only a tool as recalled by the world-renowned expert in artificial intelligence, Luc Julia. It's neither good nor bad and it really depends on what we want to do. Therefore, I felt it was important to expose some strategical use cases in order to guide current and future entrepreneurs in the field of metaverse and healthcare. This is of course a non-exhaustive list and there are still some unresolved issues and challenges. One of these challenges is user-experience which will be important for accelerating the metaverse's mass-adoption in healthcare. Many of the current users in metaverse games complain about the lack of fluidity and interoperability between 3D spaces regarding using an avatar or cryptocurrency. This problem has to be resolved before proposing any hospital, pharmacy and healthcare related initiatives. Even if the metaverse is an entry point from the real world to the virtual reality world it should be also an entry point from a metaverse to another relevant metaverse. The question of price will also be crucial for mass-adoption especially regarding the hardware part. To be honest, I continue to be concerned about the proprietary purpose of big players to this day. Which is not good for creating and developing a "fluid and affordable metaverse". I should like to conclude by alerting on many beliefs about the fact the metaverse is such a bad society where physical doctors will be replaced by AI-based avatars or where big platforms will know everything about us. This dystopia may be true for projects proposing mass-surveillance systems powered by chatbot. But I'm quite optimistic when we know that physical presence is still required for certain types of patient and medical interventions. The metaverse may not be a revolution, however, it takes us into the unknown. This book asks us: can we make health sustainable through a metaverse? The answer is yes, we can! It might be the beginning of a new world where what we do physically could also be done in a virtual reality world!

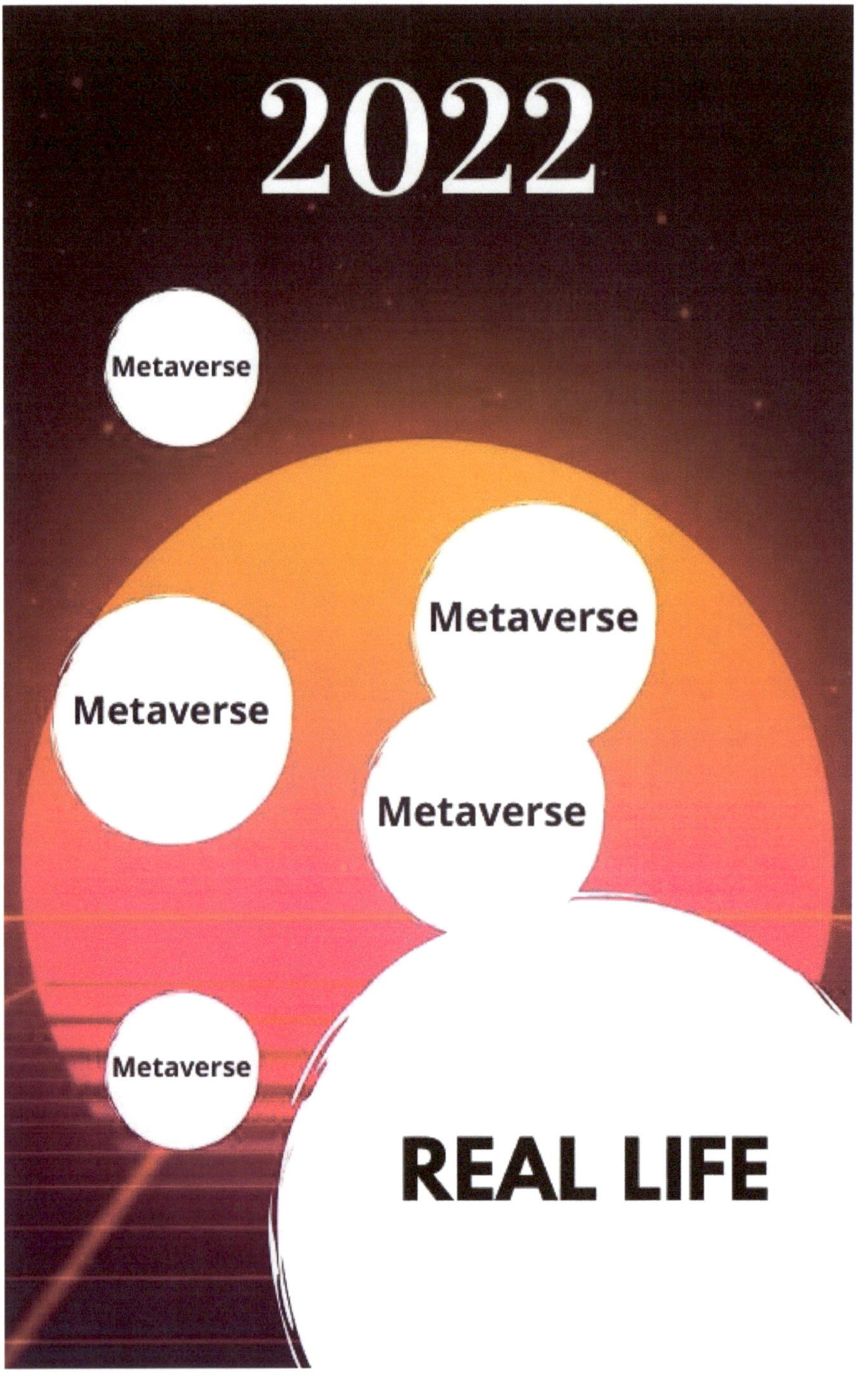

2022
Metaverse
Metaverse
Metaverse
Metaverse
Metaverse
REAL LIFE

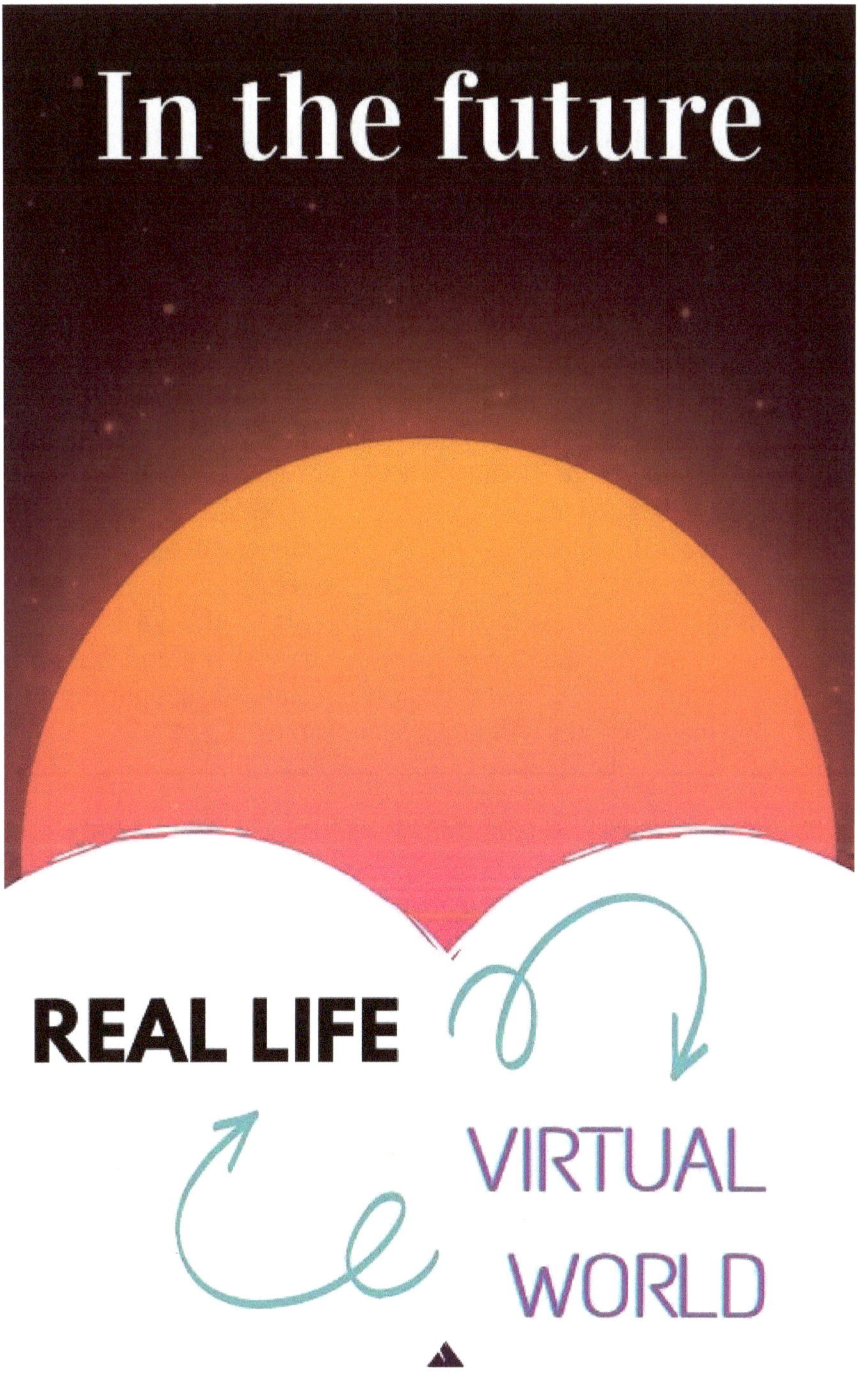

In the future
REAL LIFE
VIRTUAL WORLD

ACKNOWLEDGMENTS

I would like to thank everyone that I interviewed for sharing their insights and experiences. Whether you are named in this book or not, trust that your contribution was invaluable and that I appreciate your openness. I also want to thank my loved ones for the advice they have given me in order to make the right choice. A special thank you to my mother who was involved in the graphic design of the book. Special thanks to Ornella Fily for her profound belief in my work and constructive criticism. I'd like to acknowledge the effort of Rachel Mckinnon for her proofreading work. Thank you to Philippe Gerwill for his fantastic foresight and for always being ready to have lengthy discussion about what could deeply change the metaverse in healthcare. I also enjoyed the discussion with Luc Julia about the term of AI that has been overused for many years. "There is no such thing as Artificial Intelligence!". Last but not least, I would like to thank my European friends and collaborators for their enthusiasm about the project. Thanks for supporting me and I hope that our paths will cross again soon!

ABOUT THE AUTHOR

Lucas Perez is a medical and strategic expert in disruptive solutions for healthcare. He hosts a Youtube Webseries in partnership with an independent body of EU Commission (EIT Health Alumni) in order to popularize topics such as artificial intelligence, blockchain or longevity.

His book *Economy of Thinking* under the french title *Réussir dans l'Economie de la Pensée* and   How to Take Advantages of your Unconscious in your Daily Life? have inspired more than 10 international conferences accross Europe and Africa. And now, he's turned his attention to the incredible potential of Metaverse to create new healthcare, wellness and sport solutions.

"If you think you have an interest in navigating the digital world for your health or any reason, take it slow and don't be scared! But you should remember that sometimes history repeats itself especially in term of technology that's why
we have to place intelligence into humans above all".

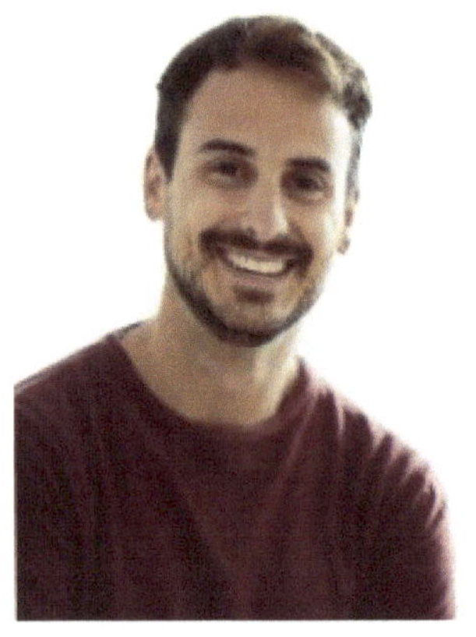

CONTENTS

INDEX